Warm Thoughts for the Heart

For New Nurses

Thoughtfully collected and written by: Anne R. Naulty, MSN, RN, PCCN

Welcome to the field of nursing! We are glad you have decided to join us! This book was written with all nurses in mind. Whether you are contemplating nursing school, in nursing school, a new graduate, a new nurse, or a nurse with experience, this book was written for you. Nurses give from their heart every day. Because of this, it is very important for us to recharge our own hearts. That is the purpose of this book. This book can be read a page a day or skimmed as needed to recharge you, a valuable nurse. It was written by nurses for nurses. It shares the knowledge and love that nurses have for each other.

Some of the information in this book was collected from nurses all over the United States. The wisdom in these pages cannot be duplicated. These nurses were asked, "What advice would you tell a new nurse (or even an experienced one)?" The information contained in this book is what these nurses have said. I added some information that I have collected over my years of teaching all nurses too! Thank you from our hearts to yours for all of the work that you do. May God bless you always.

This book is dedicated to
all people who have the
profession of
nursing in their heart.
We are the healers.

The more I see all of the suffering in the world, the more I know that I was placed in the field of nursing to make a difference. Whether it is one life that I am able to change or multiple lives, I know that I have made a difference somewhere, to someone.

Nurse's Prayer

Dear Lord, I know that I am only one, but my faith in you has made me powerful. It is through this faith, that I have learned to love others in a selfless manner. Please bless me as I comfort and assist in the healing of all of your children. May I be the voice for those who cannot speak, the strong arms for those who cannot walk, and the caring smile for those who feel alone. May I use my mind to help in the healing of my patients and may I never be silent when I need to be heard. I am blessed to be a healer. May I never take this role lightly for it is a priveldge to be able to serve others in this manner. Amen.

"I want to go to nursing school so bad, but I don't understand the process. Can you help?"

All nurses must take prerequisites before starting their nursing classes. These prerequisites, or core classes, may differ slightly depending on the institution that you choose. Prerequisites often involve chemistry, biology, anatomy, physiology, English, math, and sometimes pharmacology. There are currently two entry level degrees for nurses: the associate's degree (ASN) and the Bachelor's degree (BSN). The ASN usually takes 2-3 years to complete, while the BSN takes 4-5 years to complete. Nurses from both degrees can find jobs, however the current hospital goal is to hire more nurses with their BSN. Either way, ASN and BSN nurses can both sit for the NCLEX exam and become Registered Nurses (RN's).

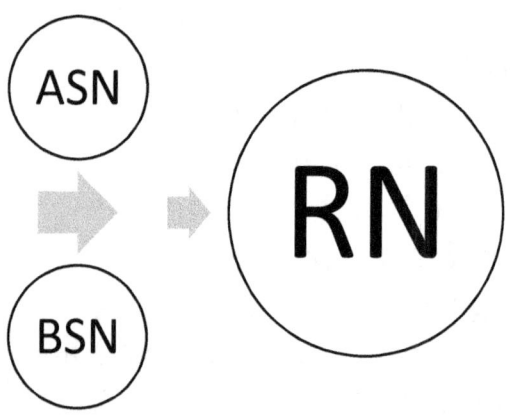

"Each person's perspective (the doctor, the patient, the nursing assistant, etc.) is equally valid and carries the same weight as your own."

~Karen, Critical Care RN, Kansas City, MO.

Learn to listen, and you will be amazed at what you learn.

Who knows the patient better than the patient? When the patient tells you something is wrong, listen to them and believe them. They know their bodies and can give the nurse more insight.

Listen to the nursing assistant. They are a nurse's best friend. They deal with the patients on a different level than the nurses do. There are times when they spend more time with the patients than the nurse. There are also times when a patient will tell the CNA something, that they do not want to tell the nurse. <u>CNA's, you are priceless.</u>

Listen to the patient's family. When they tell you something is going on, hear what they are saying. They have known this person for a long time. Learn to listen…

Take a moment for yourself…
Always take time to listen to the sounds of life and nature. Look at the sunrise and the sunset. Realize that these are all gifts from a higher power that loves and cares for us all.
Nurse recharge.

Nurses have a lot of responsibility.

This is especially true when it comes to administering medications. Sometimes the MD's will order a lot of pain medications. This does not mean that the nurse is to give them all to the patient. **Start low and move slow** is the motto. Always assess the patient before administering anything that can sedate them. It is the nurses responsibility to make discretionary calls when it comes to any 'as ordered' (prn) pain medications.

The nurse is the professional that is at the bedside and we are able to see the patient. If the patient is sedated and asking for narcotics, it is our responsibility to make the best decision for the patient.

Be open with the patient and explain your rational if possible. Assess and determine the best plan for the patient each moment. Keep flexible in this plan, and assess for the moment.

As I drive into work, I try to always take notice of the sunrise or the sunset. I tell myself, "God has made that sunrise/sunset just for me." Each one is different. Each one is beautiful. As I admire the colors, I realize that we are all part of one large being. We are all connected. We are loved. As a nurse, it is my responsibility to carry that love and give it to others. It is like I am carrying a large candle and my job is to light other people's candles so they may see the light within and around them. I show others love so that they may not only feel the love, but then they are able to give that love to others who may need it. I guess we could say that "Nurses are love."

"There are times, as a floor nurse that I feel really overwhelmed. I am trying to get my charting done and I may have a patient that continues to call out or is trying to get out of bed a lot. The bed alarms are ringing and so is my head! I know that the patient is at the center of care, but I am human too. I can only handle so much. I want to be a good nurse and care for all of my patients, but there are so many demands on us at times."

First, take a deep breath. Please understand that we all feel this way at times. An experienced nurse learns to use all of the resources that are available and to think outside of the box. It is okay to ask the other nurses in your unit for assistance so that you can get some charting done. It is also okay to take a break when you feel your head swimming. When you come back, you will probably have a different perspective. Allow yourself to be human and take a breath. Look at your feet and know that you are okay in this minute. You are loved and an important part of a large nursing family. You are not alone.

A leader is not defined by name alone. A leader is defined by the actions they take.

Leaders arise out of situtations. In healthcare, there are many opportunities for you to become the leader that you were meant to be. Continue to learn everything that you can and always look for those opportunities to help others. Always allow yourself to engage in the company that you work for and look for ways to improve the workflow. Read and learn the company vision, and mission statement and work towards that goal.

Floating to another unit can be a scary experience for any nurse. As I think back to nursing school, I remember having clinical experiences on many different units in many different hospitals. I was always nervous at first, but once I got to know the staff my comfort level would increase. I learned that it is <u>normal</u> to be nervous in new situations. I learned that it is <u>okay</u> to be nervous in new situations. In fact, it shows that we are human.

I now understand that many nurses feel nervous when they float to new units. I want to remember this nervous feeling, so I can learn to be welcoming. I want to always be one of the nurses who make the floating nurse feel comfortable. I need to figure out how to help them.

Dear God, please let me remember that everyone gets scared in new situations. I want to be the one that is able to help people to feel at ease.

"We just started to learn all of the different medications. How am I going to remember them all?"

Many years ago, there were only a few medications that medical professionals needed to know as part of their patient care. As anyone can see, the list of approved medications has increased substantially. In fact, every year when I get my new drug book, I see that it is getting thicker and thicker.

Many nurses and pharmacists suggest that learning the medications by class is the easiest method. Learn what the class does, the side effects, the mechanism of action, etc. Then notice if there are similarities in the names of the medications. An example is: many of the beta-blockers end in "olol." If you recognize this, then you will see the patterns and be able to note any differences in the individual medications from each category.

"My fear is that I will not know what to do if a patient codes. How do

nurses know what to do during these emergencies?"

Codes are not like they look in the movies. Most times, they are calm and well controlled. Medical professionals learn their code skills by taking an Advanced Cardiac class that is offered in most hospitals. These classes give the nurse the basic training that is necessary in order to participate in a code. These skills must often recertified every year or two. Once you have taken this class, you will know what to do in a code situation.

"Don't get so focused on completing your tasks that you forget that your patient is a person, and a person deserves common courtesy and respect."

~Jenny, ICU/Med Tele RN, Kansas City, MO

"Treat your patients as you would want yourself and your loved

ones to be treated (Essentially, follow the Golden Rule!) ☺
~Jane, Critical Care RN, Kanas City, MO

Don't just read these bits of wisdom, think about them for a moment:

Being a patient can be down right scary. Nurses have a great opportunity to be there for another person during this scary time. Never take that responsibility lightly. I tell all of my patients that I will treat them the way that I would treat a member of my own family and I mean it!

Give yourself the permission to not know some things. There is not a nurse alive that knows everything. The most intelligent nurses know when they need to ask for help and they do. The most dangerous nurses are the ones that think they know everything **and choose not to ask or listen to advice**.

So far, in my nursing career, everyone has taught me new things. Patients have taught me, nurses have taught me, doctors have taught me, nursing assistants have taught me, and environmental service people have taught me. I learn new things everyday from all sorts of people from all kinds of places. This is the beauty of being a nurse. Nursing uses the knowledge from so many people and from so many fields in order to give the best care to the patient.

We learn from everyone and we learn from each other. If I forget how to do something, I can ask one of my colleagues. We are always happy to help each other.

> People who are not part of the
> solution to a problem
> are, by deduction,
> part of the problem.

Choose to be part of the solution today ☺.

"I have been working on my BSN Nursing homework for hours. I am tired, and sometimes I wonder why I am doing this. Does anyone else ever wonder these things?"

As a nurse, there are so many advanced degrees and certifications that we can obtain. They are all hard work. We wear these degrees and certifications as a badge of honor and hard work. Give yourself a small pat on the back and realize that you are reaching a new level in nursing. We are <u>all cheering you on</u>! Reach FOR the stars!

Take care of yourself and you will be able to take care of others.

It is so easy to get so busy with our own lives that we neglect the most important person we know- ourself. The problem is that you cannot give to someone else, something that you do not have. In other words, you cannot give your best care, if you did not get enough sleep, have not been eating somewhat healthy, have not been drinking enough water, and have not had a little bit of fun lately! The best caregivers know this information and take it to heart. Love yourself and care for yourself. Get your regular check-ups and make time for you. We love you and know that <u>you are worth it!</u>

"Being a nurse can be expensive. We pay for many of our continuing education classes, our nursing organization dues, subscriptions, books, licensing fees, uniforms, supplies, certifications, certification renewals, and of course, advanced degrees. All of these costs start to really add up. It's tough because many hospitals are not offerring pensions, and pay raises are not as common as they once were. Place the stress that our jobs have, and sometimes I wonder

why I ever decided to do this. Does anyone ever feel this way?"

The answer is, "yes." We all feel this way at times. If you ask most nurses why they entered the profession, they will tell you that they, "wanted to help people." Many nurses will also tell you that they were called to be a nurse. This is all true. Sometimes answering a higher calling is hard and it feels like we are swimming upstream. Just remember that God will never give you more than you can handle. Trust in Him and care for his children. As you place yourself out there, He will care for you.
My Grandmother Molly (Reight) always told me that God has me in the palm of his hand. She would say that when times seemed tough, I should relax and let go. Then, and only then, would I realize how safe and loved I really was. I would know that it was really all in control.

May you feel God's love in your heart

and all around you today.

"Always use your pharmacist as a resource! It is called teamwork!"

Missy, PharmD, Overland Park, KS

There is an old African proverb that states that raising a child is not a one person job, it takes a community. This is truly the easiest and most effective manner to acomplish this task. Everybody chips in, and everyone works together. Patient care is no different. For the nurse who works in the hospital environment, the saying would be, "It takes a hospital to care for a patient." Caring for a patient involves every discipline in the hospital. Know who your resources are and ask them questions. We have all worked very hard to learn the information that we know. Ask and you will learn new things!

In times of stress and anxiety, stop and take a deep breath. Breath in ~ and breath out. Look at your feet. Realize that you are okay right in this minute. In this minute, everything is taken care of.

Take another deep breath.

Be in this minute. Breathe.

There are shifts when I have too much to do and not enough time. I can feel my blood pressure rising and I feel like I want to run away or cry. In those stressful times, I remember what my friend Nita said to me so many years ago. I stop whatever I am doing and take that deep breath. Inhale deep and long exhale. I gather my thoughts together and look at my feet. I know that I AM OKAY IN THIS MOMENT. I take another deep breath and let the oxygen flow. I AM OKAY. LIFE IS OKAY. I let the stress pass and I smile. Today is going to be a great day.

Sometimes it is the small things that we do that make the biggest difference.

Quite a few years ago, my mom suffered a major heart attack. Prior to surgery, she had a RN that seemed to bond with her. After her coronary bypass surgery (CABG), my mom was moved to the ICU. While she was recovering in the ICU, there were times that she felt very defeated. One day, this special nurse came to visit her in the ICU. She brought her a small, smooth stone and she told my mom to rub the stone when she felt sad, and then she would know that everything would be okay. She told my mother that she would know that she was loved when she rubbed this stone.

This small act of kindness touched my mother's heart in a large way. My mom says that every time that she would rub the stone, she would feel better and she would know that she was loved. That stone gave my mom the extra burst of energy to heal.

My mom, Laura, told me yesterday that she still carries this stone with her in her purse. She says that when she feels sad, she holds the small stone in her hand and rubs it with her fingers. She then begins to feel like everything will be fine and she knows that she is loved.

"If you are a new nurse, partner up with a more experienced nurse. If you are an experienced nurse, partner up with a new nurse. It is amazing how much information can be shared."
Sandi, CCU RN, Kansas City, MO

Nursing really is a team sport. There is not a nurse alive who knows everything. We teach each other as we go along. It is good to have other nurses that you feel comfortable with. Remember that it is okay to ask for help or advice. The patients are counting on it.

Nursing Organizations

There are nursing organizations in every country and in every specialty. It is always a great idea to join at least one and become active. These organizations will offer up to date knowledge in the selected specialty and they are a great place to network. Build your nursing circle and submit an abstract to the annual conference. Place yourself out there and shine! Let us get to know you!

For up to date nursing organization information, perform a search on the internet. For an annual fee, you will get the organization magazine sent to your home, you will have access to continuing education credits, you will have access to the many benefits of the website, and you will be able to show your pride in your specialization.

"Find a report sheet that works for you and use it. This way you can go to any department in the hospital or any hospital and feel comfortable. Oh ya, and don't forget to breathe."
Deb, CCU RN, Kansas City, MO

Many nurses call their report sheet their "brain," because this is the piece of paper that we write all of our patient information on. It is what we use to give and get report at shift change. It is how we organize our tasks. There are many different sheets available on the internet, however many nurses make their own. Just remember to keep it organized so that you are organized. Nursing is all about time management and organization. This is how we are able to stay on task and give the best care to all of our patients.

"Always be nice to the pharmacist."

Chris, PharmD, Arkansas

Nice to the pharmacist? Nurses are always nice to the pharmacists, aren't we? Without these important people, we are unable to accomplish the tasks at hand. We need you all, even if we do not say it! We also appreciate you. We appreciate you the most when you do a few things to help us out:

1. Don't schedule a bunch of medications at shift change.
2. Please group the medications together so we do not have to bother the patient every hour.
3. Have the medications that we need available.

Simple. Right? That is all we ask for, I think. To show how much we care for the pharmacists at our facilities, let us take a minute to give them our prayer:

"Dear Lord, please bless all of the pharmacists that work with nurses and keep them witty, quick and wise." (After all, they need to be able to keep up with us!)

"Always trust your gut and assessment skills."

Gabrielle, Obstetrics Special care nursery RN, Illinois

I feel like every time I don't trust my gut, bad things happen. If I look at something, or someone and think that something isn't right, I trust my gut and I start to take action. It does not matter that I may not have any idea what is wrong yet. I have learned to live by that rule and trust it.

"Don't take anything for granted. Always be grateful. Do your part to make a difference in this world, no matter how small the difference is. Every effort matters." Teresa, Mon Alto, PA.

Very few people enjoy being a patient. Most of the time, they don't feel well, they are tired, and they are scared. Remember that and take time to talk to your patients. They will be grateful and you will feel the difference that you make. They may forget your name, but they will remember some of the things you did for them.

Always remember that people just want to know that they matter.

Have you told someone that they matter today?

Nursing is a team effort. No one knows everything.

Nurses who think they know everything are the dangerous nurses. Information changes every day and we learn more about everything. Nursing includes so many different disciplines. Each nurse excels at a different area. Together, we are a perfect team. Never be afraid to ask a fellow nurse's opinion. We will respect you for it.

Our system is broken. You will see mistakes. You will have to fix mistakes.

Take your time when administering medication. Nurses are being made to do more and more with less resources. Nothing should ever take the place of superior patient care. I may be asked to care for more patients than I should, but I will continue to care for each one as if they were my only one. I came into nursing because I love being there for others and I want to make a difference. I will never forget that.

"Always protect yourself first. If a patient is on precautions, take the time to put on your PPE. Nothing and no one is worth getting sick over. Protect yourself first. If you don't, then who will care for the patients? Take your time when working with needles, patients with altered mental statuses, and diseases. Protect yourself." Sarah, RN, ER, San Diego, California.

Nurses deal with some of the worst diseases at times. Protect yourself and your family from the pathogens. It is always your right to wear a mask, gown, and/or gloves. You can always place a patient on precautions as a precaution. I would rather act as though someone has something and find out later that they don't have it, than assume they don't and then find out they do.

One night, I was having a tough shift on the neuroscience unit. I can't remember exactly what was going on, but I remember sitting at the computer and looking over at my coworker whose name was Friday. Friday must have sensed my mood. He came over to me, smiled, and said, "You just have to love them Anne, just love them."

That night, I learned how to open my heart and nurse with love.

Thank you Friday.

"Make today awesome for someone else. It will come back to you 100 times greater."

Monika, LPN, Columbus, OH.

"Nursing is a career that has so many specialties. Not every nurse stays at the bedside. Actually, bedside nursing is probably the hardest nursing there is. Continue to look around as see all of the different jobs that nurses have. It is one of the best careers out there. I really do believe that! I became a nurse over 25 years ago, and I have not regretted it one day since passing my NCLEX. My career has brought me to see so many things." Saundra, RN, Atlanta, Georgia.

Once you find a part of the practice you like, take the time to get certified. Certified RN's not only make a little more money, but they help their hospitals earn the Magnet status. Certification also shows that you have given that little extra effort to learn more information and pass a national test.

Invest in your profession. There are certifications for almost every area of nursing. Many times, your hospital will pay for one certification per nurse. Challenge yourself and show that you care- Earn that certification (and get more letters after your name!).

Join a nursing organization today.

There are so many nursing organizations. A simple Internet search will show you that this is true. Join an organization and slowly become active. It will help you network and expand your profession as well as your mind.

Find that organization that you feel passionate about.

Be your best.

"When I started nursing school over 50 years ago, nursing students use to have to live at a dorm that was close to the hospital. We would go to class in the morning, and then go and work at the hospital. We were under very strict rules and lived by them, or were kicked out. The MD's also worked with us and taught us while we were in the hospital. For all of the work that we did, nursing school only cost a few hundred dollars. We felt good and knew that we were making a difference in people's lives."

Marguerite, Philadelphia, PA.

"It is not about you, it is not about me, it is about the patient."

Linda, RN, Cape May, NJ.

"I have been a doctor for a long time now. I remember when I use to make house calls and charge $1.00 for my services. That dollar even included the medication that I gave to the family. I also remember when we had to increase the price for a house call to $2.00. Wow, people got upset about that one. I wonder what they would say about today's prices."

John, MD., Nevada

One night the call light went off. The nurse answered the call light, asking the patient, "Can I help you?"

"I am ready for my nightly massage," the patient replied. "It is time for me to go to sleep."

The nurse looked dumbfounded and thought that maybe she did not hear the patient right. "You are ready for your what?"

The patient replied, "I am ready for my back massage."

The nurse hung up the intercom and turned to face a more experienced nurse who was laughing. The newer nurse said, "The patient would like her massage now. What does that mean?"
The more experienced nurse then explained to the newer nurse that not too many years ago patients use to get short back rubs with moisturizer before they went to sleep. Not only did this action calm them down and loosen up their muscles, but it actually helped them sleep better.
The newer nurse looked at the older nurse, and replied,

"Now we just give them a sleeping pill."

What happened to candy stripers?

Many years ago, young people would volunteer in the hospitals. These volunteers would wear white and pink striped aprons. They were therefore called "candy stripers." There are still volunteers in every hospital, in fact we cannot live without them! These volunteers just do not have to wear the old candy striper outfits.

Thank you to all of our hospital volunteers. We appreciate you so much. May God bless you.

Hospitals are often not the way that they appear on television.

"People remember when you make them feel safe, and happy. I start each day with a prayer that I will have the opportunity to serve someone else today. I want to do God's will, and help those that are placed into my path."
　Robert, Med/Surg RN, Los Angeles, CA

"I recently had to get a uterine biopsy. After they place the scapula, they use this instrument to pull your uterus down and towards the front. At that time, I thought that I was going to jump off of the table and cry. One of the nurses who were assisting the MD, noticed my discomfort and came over and held my hand. It was amazing. All of a sudden, I did not feel so alone and scared. I am a nurse and have held many patients' hands during procedures, however I did not realize the full impact of that until this day." Anonymous

I believe that nursing is a calling and we are called into nursing by some higher power. We are the chosen healers and the keepers of the lantern. Never take this responsibility lightly. It is our responsibility to advocate for all patients so that they are able to receive the best care all of the time.

A few years ago I had a friend that was in the final stages of dying. She was on a non-rebreather. As I walked into the room and started to talk to her, she removed the oxygen and spoke back to me. She told me that she needed to write a poem for me that she felt she was supposed to give to me. I encouraged her to keep the oxygen on her face, however she said that what she had to tell me was more important. She placed the face mask back on and asked her son for a piece of paper. She told me that if I ever published a book and wanted to include it, I could include it. So, here it is:

III

A cat's paw rocking
A puppy's tail wagging
A tree silhouetted at sunset
The smell of wood smoldering
The mogie of a spider web
The world reflected in a raindrop.

Could my poor brain conceive?
By any and if these are
The existence of God's presence,
It is enough!

She was special to me and she told me that I was special to her. She truly lived life for others. She touched my heart as a person, and as a nurse. We talked on and off that night about all sorts of things. She wanted to share some of her stories with me. We both knew that she was dying, and I did everything that I could to make her comfortable. Most of all, I listened to her messages and stories as I took the time to hold her hand.

The next day I came back into the hospital to find out that my friend had passed. Her son was still there. I sat with him for a few minutes before we decided to leave the hospital.

I did not understand her message at that time, although I held on to the paper that she wrote her poem to me on all of this time. Today, I partially understand what she was trying to say and I cherish it, as I cherish her.

Take a few minutes to get to know who your patients are as people. Listen to their stories and their wisdom. It is a blessing to be able to get this close to people. Most people are wonderful and we need to celebrate them. I celebrate this wonderful woman, my friend, today.

"Nursing is not about the paperwork, it is about the people."
Janice, ICU, Florida

I remember learning in nursing school, that "if you did not chart it, you did not do it." I understand that charting is important, because it is the only record that we have which states what we did for the patient. How many hours do you spend with the patients each shift, and how many hours do you spend charting? One nurse said that she feels as if she spends 25% of her time with the patients and the rest of the time charting or looking through orders. This seems to be true, and this seems to be what nurses complain about. Somehow, someway, we need to make the charting less time consuming so that we can spend more time attending to the needs of the patients. How do we do that? I really don't know, however we are all open to suggestions.

"When you are in tough times, always remember the reason that you became a nurse. Don't give up or give in. Just shine."

Lauren, Kansas

It is okay to cry after a tough shift. As a nurse, you are still human.

TEAMWORK
Think about it.

Today is the day to inquire about a higher degree. There are so many degrees in the field of nursing. Once a nurse obtains her/his BSN, the MSN is the next step. Concentrations for MSN's include: education, leadership, informatics, and nurse practitioner.

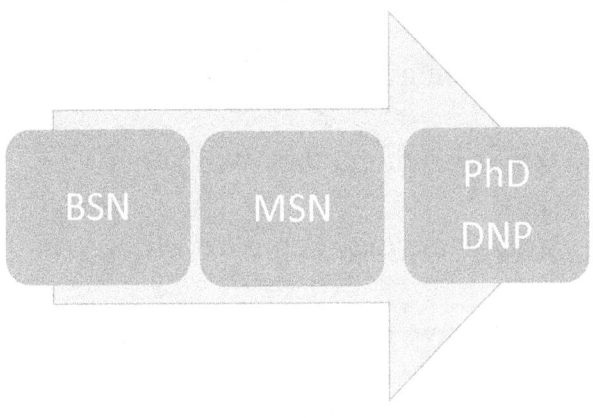

People need to know that they are being heard. Some business books call this skill "active listening," and some call it "total engagement." No matter what it is called, learn to listen without judgement and without trying to figure out how you are going to respond. People need to know that they are being heard. If they feel like no one is listening, they will get frustrated and may begin to yell.

If they have become this frustrated, affirm that you understand how they must feel and apologize for the company. Thank them for bringing the problem to your attention, and then agree on a solution. Whatever you agree on, make sure that you honor your side of the agreement. This proves that you were listening and that you care about what they said.

Never be afraid to ask the doctor questions.

Being a nurse means that you will have to have conversations with people that may make you feel a little uncomfortable. Do not be afraid to step out of your comfort zone. Patients are people and they, above anyone else, know their situation.

Don't be afraid to ask them about their religious beliefs, their families, their alcohol use, or anything else that is relevant. Having open conversations with patients is a skill that needs to be learned and practiced. It will make you a better nurse and a better person all around. If you are unsure what a person is saying, rephrase their answer and ask them if that is what they meant. Conversation is a necessary skill in nursing and must be practiced.

Always remember that humans are emotional beings. Some people are more in touch with their emotions than others, however just because someone may have difficulty expressing their emotions, does not mean that they do not have any. Don't be afraid to talk about emotions with people. Empathize with them, and encourage them to talk. Healing involves every aspect of our being. Encourage holistic healing for your patients and acknowledge their emotions.

Nurse from the

heart,

But use your mind.

As a nurse, it is important that I never stop learning. Medical knowledge and nursing practices change all of the time as we learn new things. These new practices are not going to mysteriously appear, you must seek this knowledge. As a nurse, we must **own our education**. We must always be on the look-out for better ways to care for the patients that we serve. This is part of our training, and part of the promise that we made when we became nurses.

Every business should have a vision statement, and a mission statement. The mission statement tells everyone why the business is operating. The vision statement tells the world where the business strives to go.

Today's goal: I will find out what my hospital's vision and mission statement are.

Today's goal is to create a **personal** mission and vision statement that will guide your nursing practice.

"Before you take any action, think your choice all of the way through. Some things cannot be taken back or corrected."

Matt, Pittsburgh, PA

This is true in life and in nursing. Think your way through the action before you make it. Ask yourself if the action will most likely create the desired effect.

Nursing is a profession and it is our business. It is our innate responsibility to reach the highest level that we are able to reach so that we can ultimately give the greatest good. Nurture your career and business. Prepare yourself to reach the next level (whatever that is for you).

Q: How is nursing practice changed?

A: Changing nursing practice starts with an idea of how to do a task better. The idea is then tested through research. If the research shows that the desired effect is achieved, the change can be incorporated into a theory or concept and then introduced to practice.
It all starts with an idea.

What practice would you like to change today?

Because we care for so many other people, many nurses forget to care for themselves. Take time each day to nurture yourself spiritually, mentally, physically, and socially. In order to make sure that I do this every day, I take a piece of paper and divide it into four sections. In the first section, I write "Spiritual," and I ask myself what I am going to do today to nurture myself in that section. Am I going to go to church, read the Bible, or maybe meditate? My next section of holistic development is the "mental" section. This is where I learn something new by reading, surfing the internet, or taking a new class. My third section is the "physical" section and means that I need to get up off my bottom and do something. It does not have to be an hour work-out, as a simple short walk will suffice. The last section is labeled, "social." What am I going to do today to be with other people? Some days it can mean that I call a few friends, while other days it means going out.

Today's goal is to enter yourself or a colleague in a nursing award contest.

There are so many nursing awards available to honor and recognize nurses. So far, I have been blessed to receive three of them and I have nominated many colleagues for awards. Nursing awards can be found through a simple internet search. Some of the awards are given for research achievements, and others are given to nurses who go beyond their required duties. No matter what the award is for, it is an honor to receive an award. Once you receive an award, place the name of the award on your resume and celebrate! Many times, the organization will fly the nurse to an award ceremony! Sometimes the award is given during a huge conference or dinner ceremony! No matter what, it is exciting and a gift that nurses are able to give each other just to say, "thank you."

Social Media:

Think of your nursing practice as a business. It is a business, you know? You have a license to practice, and you are hired for your skills. Because nursing is a profession that is held to the highest regard, everything we do as nurses is scrutinized. Many things we do can affect our ability to become licensed. Social media can work for us, or against us. Be careful what you post on line. Just as famous people have public relations personal, you must be your own PR representative. Make sure that anything that is out there about you is planned and shows you in a positive light. Some nurses go as far to have two separate accounts: one that states their name and is public, and the other that has a nickname and is a private listing. Even though this sounds good in practice, caution must still be taken. It only takes one person to share a personal post to bring down a career that you have worked hard to achieve. Plan the image that you want to be known for and prosper.

Conduct an internet search on yourself

today. What do you see?

I am currently pursuing my PhD in nursing leadership. In one of my classes, we are discussing the fact that everyone is born with a point of view. For some, that point of view is that of a follower and for others, the point of view is that of a leader. Leaders are able to see the entire picture and decide what needs to be changed to make the goal easier to accomplish. Leaders are often dreamers who take action. Many leaders have experienced great challenges in their lives, however they held their vision close and continued to reach for it. Great leaders do not give up because that is never an option. They realize that they must change the pathway to the goal sometimes, as this is expected. Do not be defeated by a setback. Do not give in or think that you cannot reach your goal. You can and will reach the goal if that is what you want. There are many people who will support you on this path. I am but one of those people. Do not listen to those people who tell you that you cannot or should not reach this new goal. You should and you can. Be a leader and accomplish this dream. I believe in you.

Floating to another department can be very scary for many nurses. We leave the area of care that we are used to and go to another area of the hospital. The trick that many have learned is to keep the focus on the patient. Caring for people involves the same basic skill set no matter what department you are in. If you keep your focus on the patient, then you will find that your fear decreases rapidly.

If the patient has multiple lines, then start at the patient and follow the lines back to the source. We start at the patient because this is a logical way to trace. If the patient has a nasal cannula, then trace the line back to the oxygen source. Make sure that the oxygen is on and note the settings. Is this what is charted for the patient? How is the O_2 sat? Most importantly, how does the patient look?

Once you have assessed this, then go to the next line. What is it for and what is it connected to? If you break up all of the lines in this manner, you will see that even the most complicated patient is not really as complicated as you once thought.

Remember that even the most skilled nurses become a little nervous when they float to new departments. Ask your colleagues if you have questions. Nurses help each other as needed and asked.

Many people enter nursing as a second career. This gives the profession a rich combination of talents. It is interesting to ask people what brought them into the field of nursing. The answer is often that they wanted to help people. Always remember that reason.

What brought you into the field of nursing?

"I have heard that nurses eat their young. What should I do if I am a newer nurse on a unit and there are nurses who are intimidating?"

I had a student ask me this question the other day. I actually have no idea where that phrase came from, nor do I give it much weight. The bottom line is that nurses want to take care of patients in a competent and caring manner. Some nurses are more nurturing to newer nurses than others. If the nurses see that you are caring for your patients and help others when possible, then they will all begin to warm up. In the meantime, stick with the nurses who are nurturing, but most importantly care for the patients that are assigned to you in the best way possible.

"There are so many nursing organizations. What are they all and should I join?"

Yes, there are a lot of nursing organizations. Not only are there organizations for different specialties, but there are also organizations from many different countries. If you know of a specialty that you are interested in, then as a student you are able to join at a discounted rate. If you do not know the area of nursing that you are interested in, then it is okay to wait.

  If you are in nursing school it is possible that your school offers free memberships into some national nursing organizations. Look into them by accessing their websites. Don't stress over this though. If you are a nursing student then you have enough stress going on. Concentrate on what is in front of you.

Once you graduate, nursing organizations can be a great addition to and for your practice. Organizations offer many continuing education credits, seminars, information, and a chance to mingle with other nurses in your area. Organizations also give you a great opportunity to be able to change practice for the better through research, poster presentations, and through regulations.

"I am in nursing school and I am overwhelmed. Many professors give us so much reading that it is impossible to complete all of the work. Am I really supposed to know all of the information that is in the reading assignments? If so, how am I supposed to get this all done?"

All nursing students and nurses can relate to this. Honestly, I am not sure it is possible to complete all of the reading that is assigned, however that would be ideal. If completing the reading is not possible, than scan/skim it. Find the highlighted and bolded information. Read the first sentence from each paragraph and always look at the pictures and diagrams. Once you have looked over all of the information and your notes, then go back and read anything that you are confused about. This is one of the best methods for learning a bulk of information at one time.

Information in our brains is separated into long term memory and short term memory items. When the short term items are able to be linked or converted into a long term item, we will remember the information for a long time, if not forever. It is therefore a great asset to be able to link the short term memory items to a long term memory. This helps us move the item into our long term storage and allows the

information to be learned
instead of memorized.

Please inspire me to reach higher.

People who are in the hospital are usually scared. A smile can mean more that you can ever imagine. Take time to sit with each of your patients for a few minutes at the beginning of each shift. Introduce yourself and shake their hand. Let them know that it is a pleasure to meet them. I learned this from Mary Beth, who is a great CCU nurse. At the beginning of each shift, she shakes each of her patient's hands as she introduces herself. If there is family in the room, then she introduces herself to them too. She always makes sure she updates the whiteboard in the patient's room, and writes down her direct phone number. She tells the patient that if they need anything, they can call her directly on her hospital provided phone. This helps to establish a professional healing relationship with the patient and often assists the family to have more trust in the nurse. It is really amazing to watch and a skill to remember. Thank you Mary Beth!

Now that I am a nurse, family members and friends call me and ask for advice. I even had a neighbor come over and ask me some questions about their medication. I am always careful what I say, because many times I only have a small part of the information. I refrain from giving specific advice, but I can tell them who they need to talk to. A few years ago, my mom was diagnosed with uterine cancer. I felt like all eyes were on me to monitor her care. I was a wreck and way too close to the situation to be of any use. One of my RN friends had been in a similar situation before. She turned to me one day and told me that even though I was a nurse, it was okay to be a daughter now. These words struck home. I realized that although I was a nurse, this was my mom. My love for her took priority and I could just be her daughter. I did not have to know all of the answers as that is what my colleagues were there for. Just as

I would have their family members best interests at heart, they would take care of my mom. I could just enjoy the love, and the time with my mom.

My mom and I made it through this tough time and I will never forget what my colleague said to me. When I am caring for a person whose family member is a nurse, I offer them the same words as wisdom that Hyung-He offered me. It is okay to be a daughter, son, niece, nephew, mother, father, right now.

(I love you Mom!)

As a nurse, I gain my strength from God. I ask God for the strength and the wisdom to serve Him in the best manner

possible. May I do His will always.

There are so many specialties in the hospital. In most hospitals there are many different doctors, respiratory therapists, physical therapists, occupational therapists, social workers, the iv team, environmental services, food services, etc. It is important to know that we are part of a team. No one is alone and no one can perform his/her job alone. Make sure you say "thank you" to your coworkers and stand up for them.

I believe that everyone does the best that they can with what they are given. This means that if the shift before you did not get everything done, realize that they did the best they could. None of us are perfect, and we rarely are able to get everything done. This is often not on purpose. Sometimes the nurse just needs to understand the importance of the task, or maybe they do know the importance, but they were busy with other important tasks. If this is the case, this is when the nurse can ask another nurse to assist.

Look towards the solution. Do not openly criticize your fellow nurses, instead talk to them, and educate gently. Jesus advised that those who are not perfect should not be so quick to criticize. We should gently teach each other. After all, we are all in the same profession with the same goals.

Give yourself a minute to reflect on this.

The first thing that any nurse should do when starting in a new hospital is to learn where the policies and procedures are located. The policies and procedures are the guidelines that various professionals in the hospital have created to ensure both patient and staff safety. As long as the nurse is following these procedures, he/she is covered by the hospital's legal umbrella (as long as they do not go against standard practice). Take time to become acquainted with your hospital's policies and procedures.

Also realize that since they are almost all online, sometimes the hardest part is finding the applicable policy.

Giving shift report is one of the most important tasks that we perform as a nurse. It is therefore important to organize your report through a systems approach. Many nurses start with the name of the patient, room #, age, code status, reason for admit, what happened and where patient was admitted from (home, SNF), what we are doing, what needs to be done, plan for discharge. The nurse then goes into the system's assessment: neuro (include ambulation requirements), cardiac, respiratory, GI/GU, skin, IV access (with date placed), etc. Keep it organized as you are painting a picture for the next nurse. Refrain from jumping around if possible.

One of the most powerful tools we have, is the ability to teach through storytelling. When we learn to tell stories that captivate our audience, we are able to teach lessons in a nonthreatening manner. Take a minute to think of some of the greatest storytellers in history. Who comes to mind?

My first thought is Jesus. Jesus shared stories with us that are still told today. They are stories of hope and love. The stories inspire us and call us to be our best.

As nurse leaders and healers, we hope to walk in Jesus' path by inspiring people, while teaching them about love and giving them hope. We want to inspire everyone we come in contact with. Encourage your patients and coworkers to share their stories too. We all have a story to tell.

"When I was young, I wanted to be a nurse, and when it was time, I pursued my dream. Now that I have been a nurse for a while, I realize that nursing is really not what I thought it was as a child. It has changed even in the short time that I have been a nurse. There is so much more charting to do and that is where the focus is. As a nurse, we must stay 10 steps ahead of the patient's condition, because a person's health can change in an instant. That is where our focus is. Staying attuned to our patients is not an easy task. In fact, it is often mentally, emotionally, and spiritually exhausting. It is so important that all nurses learn skills that can help them decompress and recharge. Meditation, exercising, eating right, balancing life, and staying close to God helps a lot."
Alaina, ICU, Houston, Texas

As nurses we need to talk about the good, and the bad. It is the only way that we can heal, so that we can continue to care of people. It is also important to remember that we also have to take extra special care of ourselves. We are only human.

It is okay to cry after a tough shift.

Nurses are human.

Dear Lord,

　Please bless my hands, my mind and my heart so that I may care for my patients in the best possible way today and every day.

Sincerely,

A Nurse

Thank you for taking the time to read this book. If you would like to add a quote in a possible future addition, please email me at:
Rnwithheart17@yahoo.com

May God bless you and keep you always.

Anne

www.ingramcontent.com/pod-product-compliance
Lightning Source LLC
Chambersburg PA
CBHW070258190526
45169CB00001B/463